PATHOLOGY ILLUSTRATED

Peter S. Macfarlane MB ChB FRCP(Glas) FRCP(Edin) FRCPath
Formerly Consultant Pathologist and Honorary Clinical Lecturer,
University of Glasgow at the Western Infirmary,
Glasgow, UK;
Formerly Visiting Professor of Pathology, University of California, Los Angeles, USA

Robin Reid BSc MB ChB FRCPath
Senior Lecturer and Consultant Pathologist,
University of Glasgow at the Western Infirmary,
Glasgow, UK

Robin Callander FFPh FMAA AIMI
Formerly Director, Medical Illustration Unit,
University of Glasgow, Glasgow, UK

FIFTH EDITION

CHURCHILL LIVINGSTONE
EDINBURGH LONDON NEW YORK PHILADELPHIA ST LOUIS SYDNEY TORONTO 2000

CHURCHILL LIVINGSTONE
An imprint of Harcourt Publishers Limited

First edition 1981
Second edition 1986
Third edition 1991
Fourth edition 1995
Fifth edition 2000

ISBN 0 443 05956 X

International Student Edition ISBN 0 443 05957 8

British Library Cataloguing in Publication Data
A catalogue record for this book is available from the British Library.

Library of Congress Cataloging in Publication Data
A catalog record for this book is available from the Library of Congress.

Medical knowledge is constantly changing. As new information becomes available, changes in treatment, procedures, equipment and the use of drugs become necessary. The authors and the publishers have, as far as it is possible, taken care to ensure that the information given in this text is accurate and up to date. However, readers are strongly advised to confirm that the information, especially with regard to drug usage, complies with current legislation and standards of practice.

The publisher's policy is to use **paper manufactured from sustainable forests**

Printed in China
NPC/01